GUIDE FOR ENDOMORPHS

*Understanding And Loving Your
Unique Body.With A
37 Days Sample Meal Plan.*

By

RUTH SCHWARTZH

Table of contents

Introduction:

If you're reading this, chances are you're tired of feeling like your body is a constant battleground. As an endomorph woman or man,you've likely struggled with weight management, self-doubt, and the pressure to conform to societal beauty standards. You're not alone.

For too long, the media and diet industries have perpetuated unrealistic beauty ideals, leaving many women feeling inadequate and ashamed of their bodies. But it's time to break free from these constraints and embrace your unique shape and size.

This book is your comprehensive guide to understanding and loving your endomorph body. It's a journey of self-discovery, empowerment, and practical advice to help you:

- Understand your body's unique needs and characteristics
- Develop a positive body image and self-esteem

- Create your own personalised nutrition and exercise plan
- Cultivate a supportive community and mindset
- Embrace your curves and celebrate your beauty

Throughout these pages, you'll find a mix of science, stories, and strategies to help you thrive as an endomorph woman. You'll learn how to quiet your inner critic, embrace your sensuality, and find confidence in your own skin.

Remember, your body is a temple, and it's time to treat it with love, respect, and care. You are strong, capable, and beautiful just the way you are. Let's start this journey together and embrace your curves with pride!

Chapter 1:

Understand Your Body

Discover the Science Behind Endomorph Body Types and How it Affects Your Weight, Metabolism, and Overall Health

As an endomorph woman, understanding your body is crucial to achieving optimal health and wellness. Endomorphs have a unique body composition and physiology that affects how they process food, store fat, and respond to exercise. In this chapter, we'll delve into the science behind endomorph body types and explore how it impacts your weight, metabolism, and overall health.

What is an Endomorph Body Type?

Endomorphs are one of three main body types, along with ectomorphs and mesomorphs. Endomorphs tend to have a larger bone structure, more body fat, and a slower metabolism compared to other body types. They often have a pear-shaped body, with a larger hip and thigh measurement compared to their bust and waist.

Body Composition

Endomorphs typically have a higher percentage of body fat, particularly in the hips, thighs, and buttocks. This is due to a higher number of fat cells in these areas, which can make it more challenging to lose weight and maintain weight loss.
Body Composition: Understanding the Endomorph Body

As an endomorph, your body composition plays a significant role in your overall health and wellness. Body composition refers to the proportion of fat mass to lean body mass (muscle, bone, and organs) in your body. Endomorphs tend to have a unique body composition, which can affect their weight, metabolism, and overall health.

Characteristics of Endomorph Body Composition:

1.Higher Fat Percentage: Endomorphs typically have a higher percentage of body fat, particularly in the hips, thighs, and buttocks. This can range from 25-40% body fat for women and 15-30% for men.

2. More Fat Cells: Endomorphs have a larger number of fat cells, which can make it more challenging to lose weight and maintain weight loss.

3. Larger Hip and Thigh Measurement: Endomorphs tend to have a pear-shaped body, with a larger hip and thigh measurement compared to their bust and waist.

4. Slower Metabolism: Endomorphs have a slower metabolism, meaning they burn calories at a slower rate than other body types.

5. More Muscle Mass: While endomorphs may have a higher body fat percentage, they often have more muscle mass than other body types, particularly in the lower body.

6. Water Retention: Endomorphs may experience more water retention due to hormonal fluctuations and slower digestion.

Understanding Body Fat

Body fat is essential for overall health, but excess body fat can increase the risk of chronic diseases like diabetes, cardiovascular disease, and certain types of cancer. There are two main types of body fat:

1. Subcutaneous Fat: This type of fat is stored just beneath the skin and can be measured using skinfold callipers.

2. Visceral Fat: This type of fat accumulates in the abdominal cavity and surrounds organs like the liver, intestines, and kidneys. Visceral fat is considered as one of the risk factors for chronic diseases.

Benefits of Healthy Body Composition

Maintaining a healthy body composition is important for overall health and wellness. Benefits include:

1. Improved Insulin Sensitivity

2. Enhanced Metabolism

3. Increased Energy

4. Better Digestion

5. Reduced Inflammation

6. Improved Mental Health

7. Reduced Risk of Chronic Diseases

Strategies for Improving Body Composition

1. Resistance Training: Building muscle mass through resistance training can help boost metabolism and burn fat.

2. High-Intensity Interval Training (HIIT): HIIT workouts can improve insulin sensitivity and burn fat.

3. Balanced Diet: Eating a balanced diet with plenty of protein, healthy fats, and complex carbohydrates can support weight loss and overall health.

4. Progressive Overload: Gradually increasing weight or resistance can help build muscle mass and improve body composition.

5. Adequate Sleep: Getting enough sleep is essential for hormone regulation, metabolism, and overall health.

6. Stress Management: Chronic stress can lead to increased cortisol levels, which can contribute to belly fat and poor body composition.

Metabolism

Endomorphs have a slower metabolism, meaning they burn calories at a slower rate than other body types. This can make it more difficult to lose weight and require more effort to maintain weight loss.

Hormones

Endomorphs tend to have higher levels of oestrogen and insulin, which can contribute to increased body fat and weight gain. Oestrogen promotes fat storage in the hips and thighs, while insulin regulates blood sugar levels and can contribute to weight gain when imbalanced.

Digestion

Endomorphs often have slower digestion and may experience bloating, constipation, and other digestive issues due to a slower gut motility.

Exercise and Weight Loss

Endomorphs may need to work harder to achieve weight loss due to their slower metabolism and higher body fat percentage. Resistance training and high-intensity interval training (HIIT) can be effective for endomorphs, as they help build muscle mass and boost metabolism.

Nutrition

Endomorphs may benefit from a balanced diet with plenty of protein, healthy fats, and complex carbohydrates. Avoiding processed foods, added sugars, and saturated fats can help support weight loss and overall health.

In conclusion, understanding your endomorph body type is crucial to achieving optimal health and wellness. By recognizing your unique physiology and adapting your diet and exercise routine accordingly, you can overcome the challenges associated with being an endomorph and thrive in your health journey.

Chapter 2:

Breaking Free from Societal Standards

Learn to Challenge Unrealistic Beauty Expectations and Embrace Your Unique Shape and Size

As an endomorph woman, you've likely been bombarded with societal beauty standards that perpetuate unrealistic and unattainable physical ideals. These expectations can lead to self-doubt, body shame, and a never-ending quest for an unachievable perfection. It's time to break free from these constraints and embrace your unique shape and size.

The Impact of Societal Beauty Standards

Societal beauty standards are often rooted in cultural and historical contexts, perpetuating

harmful and limiting ideals. These standards:
1. Promote unrealistic body shapes and sizes
2. Foster comparison and competition
3. Encourage dieting and disordered eating
4. Perpetuate body shaming and self-objectification
5. Limit self-expression and individuality
The Impact of Societal Beauty Standards

Societal beauty standards have a profound impact on individuals, particularly women, and can lead to:

1. Body Dissatisfaction: Constant exposure to unrealistic beauty ideals can lead to negative body image, low self-esteem, and a distorted perception of one's appearance.

2. Eating Disorders: The pressure to achieve an unattainable physical ideal can result in disordered eating, such as anorexia nervosa, bulimia nervosa, and orthorexia nervosa.

3. Mental Health Concerns: The stress of conforming to beauty standards can contribute to anxiety, depression, and other mental health issues.

4. Objectification: Reducing individuals to their physical appearance can lead to objectification, where people are seen as objects rather than whole human beings.

5. Comparison and Competition: Societal beauty standards foster a culture of comparison and competition, encouraging individuals to measure their worth against others.

6. Limited Self-Expression: Rigid beauty standards restrict personal expression and creativity, forcing individuals into narrow and conformist beauty ideals.

7. Internalised Oppression: Societal beauty standards can perpetuate systemic oppression, with marginalised groups facing additional barriers and discrimination.

8. Financial Burden: The beauty industry's emphasis on products and procedures can lead to significant financial expenditure, perpetuating consumerism and materialism.

9. Time and Energy Drain: The pursuit of beauty can consume considerable time and energy, taking away from more meaningful activities and personal growth.

10. Perpetuation of Harmful Stereotypes: Societal beauty standards often reinforce harmful gender, racial, and age-related stereotypes, perpetuating damaging social norms.

By recognizing and challenging these impacts, we can work towards a more inclusive and diverse definition of beauty, promoting self-acceptance, self-love, and individuality.

Challenging Unrealistic Beauty Expectations

Challenging unrealistic beauty expectations requires a conscious effort to reject societal norms and embrace individuality. Here are some ways to challenge these expectations:

1. Media Literacy: Critically evaluate the media you consume, recognizing photoshopped images and unrealistic beauty standards.

2. Diversify Your Feed: Follow people of different ages, sizes, races, and abilities to broaden your understanding of beauty.

3. Celebrate Imperfections: Embrace your unique features and flaws, recognizing they make you beautiful.

4. Focus on Health: Prioritise physical and mental well-being over physical appearance.

5. Speak Out: Challenge harmful beauty standards and language, promoting inclusive and respectful communication.

6. Support Inclusive Brands: Choose companies promoting diverse and realistic beauty ideals.

7. Embrace Ageing: View aging as a natural process, rejecting anti-aging stigmas and products.

8. Reject Diet Culture: Focus on nourishment and self-care, rather than restrictive dieting.

9. Redefine Beauty: Expand your definition of beauty to include qualities like kindness, intelligence, and resilience.

10. Encourage Others: Support friends and family in their self-acceptance journeys, promoting a culture of inclusivity.

11. Education and Awareness: Learn about the impact of unrealistic beauty standards and share your knowledge with others.

12. Self-Reflection: Regularly examine your own biases and beliefs, working to dismantle harmful beauty expectations.

By challenging unrealistic beauty expectations, we can create a more inclusive and accepting environment, promoting self-love and individuality. Remember, beauty is diverse, and every person deserves to feel seen and valued.

Embracing Your Unique Shape and Size

Embracing your unique shape and size is a journey of self-acceptance and self-love. It's about recognizing that your body is yours alone and celebrating its individuality. Here are some ways to embrace your unique shape and size:

1. Self-Reflection: Take time to understand your body's strengths and weaknesses, and focus on its positive aspects.

2. Let Go of Comparison: Stop comparing yourself to others, and instead, focus on your own journey.

3. Practice Self-Care: Take care of your physical and mental health by engaging in activities that bring you joy.

4. Embrace Your Curves: Celebrate your body's curves, whether they're hourglass, pear-shaped, or rectangular.

5. Find Your Personal Style: Experiment with fashion and find what makes you feel confident and comfortable.

6. Focus on Functionality: Instead of focusing on appearance, celebrate your body's capabilities and functions.

7. Surround Yourself with Positivity: Seek out supportive people who promote body positivity and self-acceptance.

8. Celebrate Your Uniqueness: Embrace your individuality and recognize that your body is a part of who you are.

Remember, your unique shape and size are a part of your identity, and embracing them is a powerful act of self-love. By accepting and celebrating your body, you'll find confidence, empowerment, and a deeper connection with yourself.

Building Body Confidence

1. Develop a growth mindset

A growth mindset is the belief that your abilities and intelligence can be developed and improved over time. When applied to body confidence, a growth mindset can help you focus on progress, not perfection. Here's how to develop a growth mindset and build body confidence:

1. Embrace Challenges: View challenges as opportunities to learn and grow, rather than threats to your ego.

2. Focus on Progress: Celebrate small victories and acknowledge the progress you've made, no matter how small.

3. Learn from Failure: Instead of dwelling on setbacks, use them as chances to learn and improve.

4. Embrace Imperfection: Recognize that nobody is perfect, and that imperfections are a natural part of the journey.

5. Practice Self-Compassion: Treat yourself with kindness and understanding, just as you would a close friend.

6. Develop Resilience: Build your ability to bounce back from difficulties and setbacks.

7. Focus on the Process: Instead of fixating on the end goal, enjoy the journey and learn from the process.

8. Seek Feedback: Ask for constructive feedback and use it as an opportunity to learn and grow.

9. Embrace Your Uniqueness: Celebrate what makes you different, and don't compare yourself to others.

10. Practice Mindfulness: Stay present and focused on the moment, without judgement.

By developing a growth mindset, you'll be able to:

- Build resilience and perseverance
- Focus on progress, not perfection
- Embrace challenges and learn from failure
- Develop a more positive body image
- Cultivate self-compassion and self-acceptance
- Embrace your uniqueness and individuality

Remember, building body confidence is a journey, and it's okay to take it one step at a time. By developing a growth mindset, you'll be better equipped to navigate the ups and downs of life with confidence and self-acceptance.

2. Focus on function over appearance

When we focus too much on our appearance, it's easy to get caught up in negative self-talk and self-criticism. Instead, try shifting your focus to what your body can do, rather than how it looks. This functional focus can help you build body confidence and appreciate your body's strengths and abilities. Here's how:

1. Celebrate Your Body's Capabilities: Make a list of all the things your body can do, from simple tasks like walking and running to more complex activities like dancing or playing sports.

2. Focus on Physical Strengths: Instead of dwelling on perceived flaws, focus on your physical strengths and abilities.

3. Practise Mindful Movement: Engage in physical activities that bring you joy, and focus on the sensations in your body as you move.

4. Embrace Your Sensuality: Celebrate your body's beauty and sexuality, and prioritise pleasure and intimacy.

5. Take Care of Your Physical Health: Focus on nourishing your body with healthy foods, staying hydrated, and getting enough sleep.

6. Try New Things: Challenge yourself to try new physical activities or sports, and celebrate your progress and growth.

7. Focus on How You Feel: Instead of fixating on how you look, focus on how you feel in your body.

8. Practice Self-Compassion: Treat yourself with kindness and understanding, just as you would a close friend.

9. Embrace Your Uniqueness: Celebrate what makes you different, and don't compare yourself to others.

10. Cultivate Gratitude: Practise gratitude for your body and its many capabilities.

By focusing on function over appearance, you'll be able to:

- Build body confidence and self-acceptance
- Appreciate your body's strengths and abilities
- Develop a more positive body image
- Cultivate self-compassion and self-love
- Embrace your uniqueness and individuality

Remember, your body is capable of amazing things. By focusing on its function and capabilities, you'll be able to build body confidence and develop a more positive and loving relationship with your body.

3.　　Practise mindful self-reflection

Mindful self-reflection is the practice of paying attention to your thoughts, feelings, and bodily sensations in the present moment, without judgement. By cultivating mindfulness, you can develop a greater awareness of your body and its needs, and build body confidence. Here's how:

1. Practice Meditation: Regular meditation can help you cultivate mindfulness and reduce self-criticism.

2. Engage in Journaling: Write down your thoughts, feelings, and bodily sensations to identify patterns and gain insight.

3. Take Self-Reflection Breaks: Take short breaks throughout the day to check in with your body and notice how you're feeling.

4.Exercise Self- Compassion Treat yourself with kindness and understanding, just as you would a close friend.

5. Challenge Negative Self-Talk: Notice when you're thinking critically about your body, and challenge those thoughts with positive, affirming ones.

6. Focus on the Present Moment: Instead of dwelling on the past or worrying about the future, focus on the present moment.

7. Cultivate Gratitude: Practise gratitude for your body and its many capabilities.

8. Embrace Imperfection: Recognize that nobody is perfect, and that imperfections are a natural part of the journey.

9. Develop Self-Awareness: Pay attention to your values, beliefs, and goals, and align them with your body confidence journey.

10. Seek Support: Surround yourself with supportive people who promote body positivity and self-acceptance.

By practising mindful self-reflection, you'll be able to:

- Develop a greater awareness of your body and its needs
- Build body confidence and self-acceptance
- Cultivate self-compassion and self-love
- Challenge negative self-talk and critical thinking
- Embrace imperfection and individuality
- Develop a more positive body image

Remember, building body confidence is a journey, and mindful self-reflection is a powerful tool to help you get there. By cultivating awareness, acceptance, and compassion, you'll be able to develop a more loving and positive relationship with your body.

4.Cultivate gratitude and appreciation

Cultivating gratitude and appreciation for your body is a powerful way to build body confidence. When you focus on what you're thankful for, you begin to see your body in a more positive light. Here's how to cultivate gratitude and appreciation:

1. Keep a Gratitude Journal: Write down three things you're thankful for about your body each day.

2. Share Your Gratitude: Express your gratitude to a friend, family member, or healthcare provider.

3. Practise Mindful Movement: Engage in physical activities that bring you joy, and focus on the sensations in your body.

4. Celebrate Your Body's Capabilities: Acknowledge and celebrate what your body can do, no matter how small it may seem.

5. Focus on Functionality: Instead of fixating on appearance, focus on what your body can do.

6. Write a Love Letter: Write a love letter to your body, expressing your gratitude and appreciation.

7. Create a Gratitude Ritual: Develop a daily or weekly ritual that cultivates gratitude, such as lighting a candle or saying a prayer.

8. Surround Yourself with Positivity: Seek out supportive people, media, and environments that promote body positivity.

9. Practice Self-Care: Take care of your physical and emotional needs, and prioritise self-care activities.

10. Embrace Your Uniqueness: Celebrate what makes you different, and don't compare yourself to others.

By cultivating gratitude and appreciation, you'll be able to:

- Build body confidence and self-acceptance
- Develop a more positive body image
- Focus on functionality and capability
- Celebrate your uniqueness and individuality
- Cultivate self-love and self-compassion
- Develop a more loving and positive relationship with your body

Remember, your body is a remarkable and capable vessel. By focusing on what you're thankful for, you'll be able to build body confidence and develop a more loving and positive relationship with your body.

5.Embrace your sensuality and sexuality

Embracing your sensuality and sexuality is an essential aspect of building body confidence. When you connect with your body's sensual and sexual nature, you cultivate a deeper appreciation and acceptance of your physical self. Here's how to embrace your sensuality and sexuality:

1. Explore Your Senses: Engage in activities that stimulate your senses, such as sensual touch, intimate massage, or erotic pleasure.

2. Practice Self-Intimacy: Take time to connect with your body, exploring your desires, needs, and boundaries.

3. Embrace Your Sexuality: Celebrate your sexual identity, orientation, and expression, and prioritise consensual and safe sexual experiences.

4. Cultivate Body Awareness: Develop awareness of your body's responses, desires, and needs, and honour them.

5. Let Go of Shame: Release societal and cultural conditioning that may lead to shame or guilt around your sensuality and sexuality.

6. Embrace Your Beauty: Celebrate your physical appearance, and recognize your beauty and attractiveness.

7. Prioritise Pleasure: Make time for activities that bring you pleasure and joy, whether solo or with a partner.

8. Communicate Your Desires: Express your needs and boundaries with confidence and assertiveness.

9. Embrace Your Femininity/Masculinity: Celebrate your gender identity and expression, and reject societal expectations that may limit your self-expression.

10. Cultivate Self-Love: Prioritise self-love, self-acceptance, and self-compassion, and recognize your worth and value.

By embracing your sensuality and sexuality, you'll be able to:

- Build body confidence and self-acceptance
- Develop a more positive body image
- Cultivate self-love and self-compassion
- Embrace your uniqueness and individuality
- Prioritize pleasure and intimacy
- Develop a more loving and positive relationship with your body

Remember, your sensuality and sexuality are a natural and beautiful part of who you are. By embracing them, you'll be able to build body confidence and develop a more loving and positive relationship with your body.

Breaking free from societal beauty standards is a journey of self-discovery and empowerment. By challenging unrealistic expectations and embracing your unique shape and size, you'll unlock a more confident, compassionate, and authentic you. Remember, your body is a temple, worthy of love, respect, and celebration. Embrace your endomorph body and shine!

Chapter 3:

Nutrition and Meal Planning for Endomorphs

As an endomorph, you have a unique body type that requires a tailored approach to nutrition and meal planning. In this chapter, we'll provide practical tips on healthy eating, portion control, and meal planning to help you achieve your weight loss and fitness goals.

Understanding Your Nutritional Needs

Endomorphs tend to gain weight easily, particularly in the hips, thighs, and buttocks. To combat this, it's essential to focus on nutrient-dense foods that promote weight loss and muscle growth. Here are some key nutritional considerations for endomorphs:

1.Macronutrient Balance: Endomorphs require a balanced diet that includes protein, carbohydrates, and healthy fats. Aim for a macronutrient breakdown of:
- 25-30% protein
- 40-50% carbohydrates
- 25-30% healthy fats

2.Protein: As an endomorph, you need adequate protein to support muscle growth and repair. Aim for 1.6-2.2 grams of protein per kilogram of body weight from sources like lean meats, fish, eggs, dairy, legumes, and plant-based options.

3.Complex Carbohydrates: Focus on complex carbs like whole grains, fruits, and vegetables, which provide sustained energy and fibre. Aim for 2-3 grams of complex carbohydrates per kilogram of body weight.

4.Healthy Fats: Include sources like nuts, seeds, avocado, and olive oil in your diet to support hormone production and overall health. Aim for 0.5-1 gram of healthy fats per kilogram of body weight.

5.Hydration: Drink plenty of water throughout the day to help control hunger and boost metabolism. Aim for at least 8-10 glasses of water per day.

6.Micronutrients: Ensure you're getting adequate vitamins and minerals through your diet or supplements. Key micronutrients for endomorphs include:
  - Vitamin D
  - Omega-3 fatty acids
  - Magnesium
  - Potassium

7.Caloric Intake: As an endomorph, you may need to adjust your caloric intake based on your activity level and weight loss goals. Aim for a caloric deficit of 500-1000 calories per day to support weight loss.

8.Meal Frequency: Eat frequent, balanced meals to maintain stable energy levels and control hunger. Aim for 4-6 main meals and 2-3 snacks per day.

9.Portion Control: Use a food scale or measuring cups to gauge your portion sizes and avoid overeating.

10.Individual Needs: Remember that everyone's nutritional needs are different. Be sure to consult with a healthcare professional or registered dietitian to determine the best nutrition plan for your specific needs.

Healthy Eating Tips

As an endomorph, you have a unique body type that requires a tailored approach to healthy eating. Here are some additional tips to support your weight loss and fitness goals:

1.Eat Protein-Rich Foods: Protein takes more energy to digest, which can help increase your metabolism and support weight loss. Aim for protein-rich foods like lean meats, fish, eggs, dairy, legumes, and plant-based options.

2.Incorporate Healthy Fats: Healthy fats like avocado, nuts, and olive oil support hormone production and can help you feel full and satisfied.

3.Choose Complex Carbohydrates: Whole grains, fruits, and vegetables provide sustained energy and fibre, which can help regulate blood sugar levels and support weight loss.

4.Watch Your Portion Sizes: Endomorphs tend to gain weight easily, so it's essential to control your portion sizes to maintain a healthy caloric intake.

5. Eat Frequent, Balanced Meals: Space out your meals every 3-4 hours to maintain stable energy levels and control hunger.

6.Limit Processed Foods: Processed foods are often high in added sugars, salt, and unhealthy fats, which can hinder weight loss and overall health.

7.Stay Hydrated: Drink plenty of water throughout the day to help control hunger and boost metabolism.

8.Be Mindful of Your Macronutrient Balance: Aim for a balanced diet that includes protein, carbohydrates, and healthy fats in the right proportions for your body type.

9.Incorporate Fermented Foods: Fermented foods like kimchi, sauerkraut, and yoghourt contain probiotics, which can support gut health and immune function.

10.Consult with a Healthcare Professional or Registered Dietitian: Everyone's nutritional needs are different, so it's essential to work with a healthcare professional or registered dietitian to determine the best nutrition plan for your specific needs.

Remember, healthy eating is just one aspect of a balanced lifestyle. Combine these tips with regular exercise and stress management techniques to support your overall health and wellness journey.

Meal Planning

As an endomorph, you have a unique body type that requires a tailored approach to meal planning. Your body tends to store fat easily, particularly in the hips, thighs, and buttocks, and you may struggle with weight loss. However, with a well-structured meal plan, you can support your weight loss goals and maintain overall health.

Breakfast

Breakfast is the most important meal of the day, and as an endomorph, you want to make sure you're fueling your body with the right nutrients. Aim for a balanced breakfast that includes protein, complex carbohydrates, and healthy fats. Here are some breakfast ideas:

- Oatmeal with fruit and nuts
- Greek yoghourt with berries and honey
- Scrambled eggs with whole wheat toast and avocado
- Smoothie bowl with protein powder, spinach, banana, and almond milk topped with nuts and seeds

Lunch

Lunch should be a balanced meal that includes protein, complex carbohydrates, and healthy fats. Aim for a meal that's around 400-500 calories. Here are some lunch ideas:

- Grilled chicken breast with quinoa and steamed vegetables
- Whole wheat pita with roasted turkey breast, avocado, and mixed greens

- Lentil soup with whole wheat bread and a side salad
- Grilled salmon with brown rice and sautéed spinach

Dinner

Dinner should be a balanced meal that includes protein, complex carbohydrates, and healthy fats. Aim for a meal that's around 500-600 calories. Here are some dinner ideas:

- Grilled chicken breast with roasted sweet potatoes and steamed broccoli
- Baked salmon with quinoa and sautéed asparagus
- Turkey and vegetable stir-fry with brown rice
- Grilled turkey burger on a whole wheat bun with avocado and sweet potato fries

Snacks

Snacks are important to keep you full and satisfied between meals. Aim for snacks that are around 100-200 calories. Here are some snack ideas:

- Fresh fruit and nuts
- Greek yoghourt with honey and almonds
- Hard-boiled eggs
- Carrot sticks with hummus

Tips for Staying on Track

1.Plan your meals: Take some time each week to plan out your meals for the next few days. This will help you stay on track and avoid last-minute unhealthy choices.

2.Shop smart: Make a grocery list and stick to it. Avoid buying processed and high-calorie foods.

3.Cook at home: Cooking at home allows you to control the ingredients and portion sizes. Aim to cook at home most nights of the week.

4.Stay hydrated: Drink plenty of water throughout the day to help control hunger and boost metabolism.

5.Be mindful of portion sizes: Endomorphs tend to gain weight easily, so it's essential to control your portion sizes to maintain a healthy caloric intake.

6.*Eat slowly and mindfully:* Take your time when eating and pay attention to your hunger and fullness cues.

7.*Get enough sleep:* Lack of sleep can increase hunger and cravings for unhealthy foods. Aim for 7-9 hours of sleep per night.

37 DAYS MEAL PLAN

Day 1

Breakfast: Oatmeal with banana, almond butter, and a splash of low-fat milk (300 calories)
- Snack: Apple slices with a tablespoon of peanut butter (150 calories)

Lunch: Grilled chicken breast with quinoa and steamed vegetables (400 calories)
- Snack: Greek yoghourt with berries and a sprinkle of granola (150 calories)

Dinner: Baked salmon with sweet potato and green beans (500 calories)

Day 2

Breakfast: Scrambled eggs with whole wheat toast and a slice of avocado (250 calories)
- Snack: Carrot sticks with hummus (100 calories)

Lunch: Turkey and avocado wrap with mixed greens (450 calories)
- Snack: Rice cakes with almond butter and banana slices (150 calories)

Dinner: Grilled chicken breast with brown rice and steamed broccoli (500 calories)

Day 3

Breakfast: Smoothie bowl with protein powder, spinach, banana, and almond milk topped with nuts and seeds (350 calories)
- Snack: Hard-boiled egg and cherry tomatoes (100 calories)

Lunch: Lentil soup with whole wheat bread and a side salad (450 calories)
- Snack: Cottage cheese with cucumber slices (150 calories)

Dinner: Grilled turkey burger on a whole wheat bun with avocado and sweet potato fries (550 calories)

Day 4

Breakfast: Greek yogurt with honey and mixed berries (200 calories)
- Snack: Protein bar (120 calories)

Lunch: Grilled chicken Caesar salad (400 calories)
- Snack: Apple slices with a tablespoon of almond butter (150 calories)

Dinner: Baked chicken breast with quinoa and steamed asparagus (500 calories)

Day 5

Breakfast: Avocado toast on whole wheat bread with scrambled eggs (300 calories)

- Snack: Rice crackers with hummus (150 calories)

Lunch: Grilled chicken wrap with mixed greens and whole wheat tortilla (450 calories)
- Snack: Greek yoghourt with mixed berries and a sprinkle of granola (150 calories)

Dinner: Grilled salmon with brown rice and steamed green beans (500 calories)

Day 6

Breakfast: Omelette with vegetables and whole wheat toast (250 calories)
- Snack: Carrot sticks with hummus (100 calories)

Lunch: Turkey and cheese sandwich on whole wheat bread with a side salad (500 calories)
- Snack: Apple slices with a tablespoon of peanut butter (150 calories)

Dinner: Grilled chicken breast with roasted vegetables and quinoa (550 calories)

Day 7

Breakfast: Breakfast burrito with scrambled eggs, black beans, and avocado (350 calories)
- Snack: Protein smoothie with banana and almond milk (200 calories)

Lunch: Grilled chicken Caesar salad (400 calories)
- Snack: Rice crackers with hummus (150 calories)

Dinner: Baked chicken breast with sweet potato and steamed broccoli (500 calories)

Day 8

Breakfast: Oatmeal with berries and almond milk (300 calories, 30g protein)
- Snack: Greek yoghourt with nuts and seeds (150 calories, 10g protein)

Lunch: Grilled chicken breast with quinoa and vegetables (400 calories, 40g protein)
- Snack: Apple slices with peanut butter (150 calories, 8g protein)

Dinner: Baked salmon with sweet potato and green beans (400 calories, 35g protein)

Day 9

Breakfast: Scrambled eggs with spinach and whole wheat toast (250 calories, 20g protein)
- Snack: Cottage cheese with cucumber slices (150 calories, 20g protein)

Lunch: Turkey and avocado wrap with mixed greens (500 calories, 35g protein)
- Snack: Carrot sticks with hummus (100 calories, 5g protein)

Dinner: Grilled turkey burger with brown rice and steamed broccoli (500 calories, 30g protein)

Day 10

Breakfast: Smoothie bowl with protein powder, banana, spinach, and almond milk (350 calories, 25g protein)
- Snack: Hard-boiled egg and cherry tomatoes (100 calories, 6g protein)

Lunch: Grilled chicken breast with brown rice and mixed vegetables (400 calories, 35g protein)
- Snack: Rice cakes with almond butter and banana slices (150 calories, 8g protein)

Dinner: Slow-cooked lentil soup with whole grain bread (400 calories, 20g protein)

Day 11

Breakfast: Greek yogurt with berries and granola (300 calories, 20g protein)
- Snack: Protein smoothie with banana, spinach, and almond milk (200 calories, 25g protein)

Lunch: Grilled chicken breast with quinoa and steamed asparagus (400 calories, 35g protein)
- Snack: Cucumber slices with hummus (100 calories, 5g protein)

Dinner: Baked cod with brown rice and sautéed vegetables (400 calories, 30g protein)

Day 12

Breakfast: Avocado toast on whole grain bread with scrambled eggs (350 calories, 20g protein)
- Snack: Carrot sticks with almond butter (150 calories, 8g protein)

Lunch: Turkey and cheese salad with mixed greens and whole grain crackers (500 calories, 30g protein)
- Snack: Apple slices with cheddar cheese (150 calories, 10g protein)

Dinner: Grilled shrimp with quinoa and steamed green beans (400 calories, 20g protein)

Day 13

Breakfast: Omelette with mushrooms, spinach, and whole wheat toast (300 calories, 20g protein)
- Snack: Rice cakes with peanut butter and banana slices (150 calories, 8g protein)

Lunch: Grilled chicken breast with brown rice and mixed vegetables (400 calories, 35g protein)

- Snack: Protein bar (150 calories, 10g protein)

Dinner: Slow-cooked chicken stew with whole grain bread (400 calories, 30g protein)

Day 14

Breakfast: Whole grain waffles with scrambled eggs and mixed berries (300 calories, 20g protein)
- Snack: Greek yogurt with honey and mixed nuts (150 calories, 10g protein)

Lunch: Grilled chicken breast with roasted sweet potatoes and steamed Brussels sprouts (400 calories, 35g protein)
- Snack: Carrot and celery sticks with hummus (100 calories, 5g protein)

Dinner: Baked salmon with quinoa and sautéed spinach (400 calories, 30g protein)

Day 15

Breakfast: Smoothie bowl with protein powder, banana, almond milk, and almond butter topping (350 calories, 25g protein)

- Snack: Hard-boiled egg and cherry tomatoes (100 calories, 6g protein)

Lunch: Turkey and avocado wrap with mixed greens and whole wheat tortilla (500 calories, 30g protein)
- Snack: Cucumber slices with dill dip (100 calories, 5g protein)

Dinner: Grilled pork tenderloin with roasted broccoli and brown rice (400 calories, 30g protein)

Day 16

Breakfast: Whole grain toast with almond butter and sliced banana (300 calories, 8g protein)
- Snack: Protein bar (150 calories, 10g protein)

Lunch: Grilled chicken Caesar salad with whole wheat croutons (400 calories, 30g protein)
- Snack: Rice cakes with almond butter and banana slices (150 calories, 8g protein)

Dinner: Slow-cooked beef stew with whole grain bread (400 calories, 30g protein)

Day 17

Breakfast: Whole grain pancakes with scrambled turkey sausage and mixed berries (350 calories, 25g protein)
- Snack: Greek yogurt with mixed nuts and honey (150 calories, 10g protein)

Lunch: Grilled chicken breast with roasted asparagus and quinoa (400 calories, 35g protein)
- Snack: Carrot and celery sticks with hummus (100 calories, 5g protein)

Dinner: Baked cod with brown rice and steamed green beans (400 calories, 30g protein)

Day 18

Breakfast: Smoothie bowl with protein powder, banana, almond milk, and almond butter topping (350 calories, 25g protein)
- Snack: Hard-boiled egg and cherry tomatoes (100 calories, 6g protein)

Lunch: Turkey and cheese sandwich on whole wheat bread with a side of mixed greens (500 calories, 30g protein)
- Snack: Cucumber slices with dill dip (100 calories, 5g protein)

Dinner: Grilled shrimp with quinoa and sautéed bell peppers (400 calories, 20g protein)

Day 19

Breakfast: Whole grain waffles with scrambled eggs and mixed berries (300 calories, 20g protein)
- Snack: Protein bar (150 calories, 10g protein)

Lunch: Grilled chicken Caesar salad with whole wheat croutons (400 calories, 30g protein)
- Snack: Rice cakes with almond butter and banana slices (150 calories, 8g protein)

Dinner: Slow-cooked chicken stew with whole grain bread (400 calories, 30g protein)

Day 20

Breakfast: Whole grain French toast with scrambled eggs and mixed berries (350 calories, 20g protein)
- Snack: Greek yogurt with honey and mixed nuts (150 calories, 10g protein)

Lunch: Grilled chicken breast with roasted carrots and brown rice (400 calories, 35g protein)
- Snack: Cucumber slices with hummus (100 calories, 5g protein)

Dinner: Baked salmon with quinoa and steamed broccoli (400 calories, 30g protein)

Day 21

Breakfast: Smoothie bowl with protein powder, banana, almond milk, and almond butter topping (350 calories, 25g protein)
- Snack: Hard-boiled egg and cherry tomatoes (100 calories, 6g protein)

Lunch: Turkey and avocado wrap with mixed greens and whole wheat tortilla (500 calories, 30g protein)

- Snack: Carrot and celery sticks with hummus (100 calories, 5g protein)

Dinner: Grilled pork tenderloin with roasted Brussels sprouts and sweet potatoes (400 calories, 30g protein)

Day 22

Breakfast: Whole grain oatmeal with scrambled eggs and mixed berries (300 calories, 20g protein)
- Snack: Protein bar (150 calories, 10g protein)

Lunch: Grilled chicken breast with mixed greens and whole wheat pita (400 calories, 30g protein)
- Snack: Rice cakes with almond butter and banana slices (150 calories, 8g protein)

Dinner: Slow-cooked beef stew with whole grain bread (400 calories, 30g protein)

Day 23

Breakfast: Whole grain cereal with almond milk, banana, and scrambled eggs (350 calories, 20g protein)

- Snack: Greek yoghourt with mixed berries and honey (150 calories, 10g protein)

Lunch: Grilled chicken breast with roasted bell peppers and quinoa (400 calories, 35g protein)
- Snack: Carrot and celery sticks with hummus (100 calories, 5g protein)

Dinner: Baked cod with brown rice and steamed asparagus (400 calories, 30g protein)

Day 24

Breakfast: Smoothie bowl with protein powder, spinach, almond milk, and almond butter topping (350 calories, 25g protein)
- Snack: Hard-boiled egg and cherry tomatoes (100 calories, 6g protein)

Lunch: Turkey and cheese salad with mixed greens, whole wheat crackers, and avocado (500 calories, 30g protein)
- Snack: Cucumber slices with dill dip (100 calories, 5g protein)

Dinner: Grilled shrimp with quinoa and sautéed mushrooms (400 calories, 20g protein)

Day 25

Breakfast: Whole grain toast with scrambled eggs, avocado, and cherry tomatoes (300 calories, 20g protein)
- Snack: Protein bar (150 calories, 10g protein)

Lunch: Grilled chicken Caesar salad with whole wheat croutons (400 calories, 30g protein)
- Snack: Rice cakes with almond butter and banana slices (150 calories, 8g protein)

Dinner: Slow-cooked chicken stew with whole grain bread (400 calories, 30g protein)

Day 26

Breakfast: Whole grain waffles with scrambled turkey sausage and mixed berries (350 calories, 25g protein)

- Snack: Greek yogurt with honey and mixed nuts (150 calories, 10g protein)

Lunch: Grilled chicken breast with roasted sweet potatoes and steamed green beans (400 calories, 35g protein)
- Snack: Carrot and celery sticks with hummus (100 calories, 5g protein)

Dinner: Baked salmon with quinoa and sautéed spinach (400 calories, 30g protein)

Day 27

Breakfast: Smoothie bowl with protein powder, banana, almond milk, and almond butter topping (350 calories, 25g protein)
- Snack: Hard-boiled egg and cherry tomatoes (100 calories, 6g protein)

Lunch: Turkey and avocado wrap with mixed greens and whole wheat tortilla (500 calories, 30g protein)
- Snack: Cucumber slices with dill dip (100 calories, 5g protein)
Dinner: Grilled pork tenderloin with roasted Brussels sprouts and brown rice (400 calories, 30g protein)

Day 28

Breakfast: Whole grain French toast with scrambled eggs and mixed berries (350 calories, 20g protein)
- Snack: Protein bar (150 calories, 10g protein)

Lunch: Grilled chicken breast with mixed greens and whole wheat pita (400 calories, 30g protein)
- Snack: Rice cakes with almond butter and banana slices (150 calories, 8g protein)

Dinner: Slow-cooked beef stew with whole grain bread (400 calories, 30g protein)

Day 29

Breakfast: Whole grain oatmeal with scrambled eggs, banana, and almond butter (350 calories, 20g protein)
- Snack: Greek yoghourt with mixed berries and honey (150 calories, 10g protein)

Lunch: Grilled chicken breast with roasted carrots and quinoa (400 calories, 35g protein)

- Snack: Carrot and celery sticks with hummus (100 calories, 5g protein)

Dinner: Baked cod with brown rice and steamed broccoli (400 calories, 30g protein)

Day 30

Breakfast: Smoothie bowl with protein powder, spinach, almond milk, and almond butter topping (350 calories, 25g protein)
- Snack: Hard-boiled egg and cherry tomatoes (100 calories, 6g protein)

Lunch: Turkey and cheese salad with mixed greens, whole wheat crackers, and avocado (500 calories, 30g protein)
- Snack: Cucumber slices with dill dip (100 calories, 5g protein)

Dinner: Grilled shrimp with quinoa and sautéed asparagus (400 calories, 20g protein)

Day 31

Breakfast: Whole grain toast with scrambled eggs, avocado, and cherry tomatoes (300 calories, 20g protein)

- Snack: Protein bar (150 calories, 10g protein)

Lunch: Grilled chicken Caesar salad with whole wheat croutons (400 calories, 30g protein)
- Snack: Rice cakes with almond butter and banana slices (150 calories, 8g protein)

Dinner: Slow-cooked chicken stew with whole grain bread (400 calories, 30g protein)

Day 32

Breakfast: Whole grain waffles with scrambled turkey sausage, mixed berries, and yoghourt (350 calories, 25g protein)
- Snack: Apple slices with almond butter (150 calories, 8g protein)

Lunch: Grilled chicken breast with roasted bell peppers, quinoa, and avocado (400 calories, 35g protein)
- Snack: Carrot and celery sticks with hummus (100 calories, 5g protein)

*Dinner:*Baked salmon with sweet potatoes and steamed green beans (400 calories, 30g protein)

Day 33

Breakfast: Smoothie bowl with protein powder, banana, almond milk, and almond butter topping (350 calories, 25g protein)
- Snack: Hard-boiled egg and cherry tomatoes (100 calories, 6g protein)

Lunch: Turkey and cheese wrap with mixed greens, whole wheat tortilla, and avocado (500 calories, 30g protein)
- Snack: Cucumber slices with dill dip (100 calories, 5g protein)

Dinner: Grilled pork tenderloin with roasted Brussels sprouts and brown rice (400 calories, 30g protein)

Day 34

Breakfast: Whole grain French toast with scrambled eggs, mixed berries, and yogurt (350 calories, 20g protein)

- Snack: Protein bar (150 calories, 10g protein)

Lunch: Grilled chicken breast with mixed greens and whole wheat pita (400 calories, 30g protein)
- Snack: Rice cakes with almond butter and banana slices (150 calories, 8g protein)

Dinner: Slow-cooked beef stew with whole grain bread (400 calories, 30g protein)

Day 35

Breakfast: Whole grain oatmeal with scrambled eggs, banana, and honey (350 calories, 20g protein)
- Snack: Greek yoghourt with mixed berries and nuts (150 calories, 10g protein)

Lunch: Grilled chicken breast with roasted carrots, quinoa, and avocado (400 calories, 35g protein)
- Snack: Carrot and celery sticks with hummus (100 calories, 5g protein)

Dinner: Baked cod with brown rice and steamed broccoli (400 calories, 30g protein)

Day 36

Breakfast: Smoothie bowl with protein powder, spinach, almond milk, and almond butter topping (350 calories, 25g protein)
- Snack: Hard-boiled egg and cherry tomatoes (100 calories, 6g protein)

Lunch: Turkey and cheese salad with mixed greens, whole wheat crackers, and avocado (500 calories, 30g protein)
- Snack: Cucumber slices with dill dip (100 calories, 5g protein)

Dinner: Grilled shrimp with quinoa and sautéed asparagus (400 calories, 20g protein)

Day 37

Breakfast: Whole grain toast with scrambled eggs, avocado, and cherry tomatoes (300 calories, 20g protein)
- Snack: Protein bar (150 calories, 10g protein)
Lunch: Grilled chicken Caesar salad with whole wheat croutons (400 calories, 30g protein)

- Snack: Rice cakes with almond butter and banana slices (150 calories, 8g protein)

Dinner: Slow-cooked chicken stew with whole grain bread (400 calories, 30g protein)

This meal plan provides approximately 1700-1800 calories per day, with a balance of protein, healthy fats, and complex carbohydrates to support weight loss and overall health for an endomorph. However, this is just a sample meal plan, and you should adjust the portion sizes and food choices based on your individual needs and preferences. Also, make sure to drink plenty of water throughout the day to stay hydrated!

Nutrition and meal planning are critical components of a successful weight loss and fitness journey for endomorphs. By focusing on nutrient-dense foods, controlling portion sizes, and meal planning, you'll be able to achieve your goals and maintain a healthy, balanced lifestyle. Remember to stay hydrated, listen to your body, and make adjustments as needed to ensure you're fueling your body for optimal performance.

Chapter 4:

Effective Exercise and Movement

As an endomorph, it's essential to incorporate physical activity into your daily routine to support weight loss and overall health. Exercise not only burns calories but also helps build muscle mass, which further enhances metabolism. In this chapter, we'll discuss effective exercise and movement strategies tailored to endomorphs.

Understanding Your Body Type

Before starting any exercise program, it's crucial to understand your body type and its unique characteristics. Endomorphs tend to store fat easily, particularly in the hips, thighs, and buttocks. Therefore, it's essential to focus on exercises that target these areas and promote overall weight loss.

Cardiovascular Exercise

Cardiovascular exercise is an excellent way to burn calories and improve cardiovascular health. As an endomorph, aim for at least 150 minutes of moderate-intensity aerobic exercise per week. Some effective cardio exercises include:

- Brisk walking
- Jogging or running
- Swimming
- Cycling
- Dancing

Resistance Training

Resistance training helps build muscle mass, which is essential for endomorphs. Focus on exercises that target multiple muscle groups at once, such as:

- Squats
- Lunges
- Deadlifts
- Bench press
- Rows

High-Intensity Interval Training (HIIT)

HIIT involves short bursts of high-intensity exercise followed by brief periods of rest. This type of training is ideal for endomorphs as it promotes weight loss and improves insulin sensitivity. Examples of HIIT workouts include:

- Sprint intervals
- Burpees
- Jump squats
- Mountain climbers
- Plank jacks

Core Strength

Core strength is essential for overall stability and balance. As an endomorph, focus on exercises that target your core muscles, such as:

- Planks
- Russian twists
- Leg raises
- Bicycle crunches
- Pallof press

Flexibility and Stretching

Flexibility and stretching exercises help improve range of motion and reduce injury risk. As an endomorph, incorporate stretching exercises into your routine, such as:

- Hamstring stretches
- Hip flexor stretches
- Quad stretches
- Chest stretches
- Shoulder rolls

Progressive Overload

Progressive overload involves gradually increasing the intensity of your workouts by adding weight, reps, or sets over time. This is essential for endomorphs to continue challenging their muscles and promoting weight loss.

Sample Workout Routine

Below is a sample a workout routine :

Monday (Cardio Day)

- 30-minute brisk walk or jog
- 10-minute stretching

Tuesday (Upper Body Day)

- Push-ups (3 sets of 12 reps)
- Incline dumbbell press (3 sets of 12 reps)
- Bent-over dumbbell rows (3 sets of 12 reps)
- Tricep dips (3 sets of 12 reps)
- Bicep curls (3 sets of 12 reps)

Wednesday (Rest Day)

Thursday (Lower Body Day):

- Squats (3 sets of 12 reps)
- Romanian deadlifts (3 sets of 12 reps)
- Calf raises (3 sets of 12 reps)
- Lunges (3 sets of 12 reps per leg)
- Leg press (3 sets of 12 reps)

Friday (Cardio Day):

- 30-minute cycling or swimming

- 10-minute stretching

Saturday and Sunday (Rest Days)

Remember to adjust the intensity and volume of your workouts based on your individual needs and progress. It's also essential to consult with a healthcare professional or certified personal trainer to ensure a safe and effective exercise program.

Chapter 5:

Mindset Shifts and Self-Care

As an endomorph, it's essential to focus on both physical and mental well-being to achieve optimal health and weight loss. In this chapter, we'll explore the importance of mindset shifts and self-care practices to support your journey.

Mindset Shifts

1.Embrace Your Body Type: Accept and love your body type, rather than trying to change it to fit an unrealistic ideal.

2.Focus on Progress, Not Perfection: Celebrate small victories and acknowledge progress, rather than striving for perfection.

3.Practice Self-Compassion: Treat yourself with kindness, understanding, and patience, just as you would a close friend.

4.Reframe Negative Self-Talk: Challenge negative thoughts and replace them with positive, empowering affirmations.

5.Embrace Imperfection: Recognize that nobody is perfect, and it's okay to make mistakes.

Self-Care Practices

1.Mindfulness and Meditation: Regular mindfulness and meditation practice can help reduce stress and increase self-awareness.
2.Journaling: Write down your thoughts, feelings, and gratitudes to process emotions and reflect on progress.
3.Grounding Techniques: Use sensory experiences like deep breathing, walking, or creative activities to ground yourself in the present moment.
4.Boundary Setting: Establish healthy boundaries with others to protect your time, energy, and emotional well-being.
5.Pampering and Relaxation: Treat yourself to activities that bring joy and relaxation, such as reading, taking a bath, or getting a massage.
6.Social Support: Surround yourself with positive, supportive people who encourage and uplift you.

7.Self-Reflection and Self-Awareness: Regularly examine your thoughts, feelings, and actions to gain insight and make positive changes.

8.Creative Expression: Engage in creative activities like art, music, or writing to express emotions and tap into your creative potential.

9.Nature Connection: Spend time in nature to reduce stress, improve mood, and increase feelings of connection and wonder.

10.Self-Forgiveness and Self-Love: Practice self-forgiveness and self-love by treating yourself with kindness, understanding, and compassion.

Sample Self-Care Routine

Here's a sample self-care routine to get you started:

Monda

- 10-minute morning meditation
- Journaling before bed

Tuesday

- 30-minute walk during lunch break
- Creative activity (drawing, painting, or writing) for 30 minutes

Wednesday

- 10-minute deep breathing exercise
- Reading for 30 minutes before bed

Thursday

- 30-minute yoga or stretching
- Gratitude journaling before bed

Friday

- 10-minute mindfulness exercise
- Relaxing bath or shower before bed

Saturday

- 60-minute nature walk or hike
- Creative activity (photography, gardening, or cooking) for 60 minutes

Sunday

- 30-minute self-reflection and journaling
- Pampering activity (massage, facial, or manicure) for 60 minutes

Remember, self-care is not a one-size-fits-all approach.Experiment with different activities and find what works best for you and your unique needs. By incorporating mindset shifts and self-care practices into your daily routine, you'll be better equipped to handle challenges, stay motivated, and achieve your goals.

Chapter 6:

Overcoming Emotional Eating

As an endomorph, you may have struggled with emotional eating, using food as a coping mechanism for stress, anxiety, or other emotions. This chapter will help you understand the connection between emotions and eating, and provide practical strategies to overcome emotional eating.

Understanding Emotional Eating

Emotional eating is a complex phenomenon that involves using food as a coping mechanism for emotional distress. It's a common struggle for many individuals, particularly endomorphs, who may turn to food for comfort, stress relief, or to fill emotional voids. To overcome emotional eating, it's essential to understand its underlying causes, signs, and consequences.

Causes of Emotional Eating

1.Emotional Trauma: Past experiences, such as childhood abuse, neglect, or loss, can lead to emotional eating as a coping mechanism.

2.Stress and Anxiety: Modern life's fast pace and pressure can trigger emotional eating as a way to temporarily escape or calm down.

3.Low Self-Esteem: Negative self-image and self-doubt can lead to using food as a source of comfort and validation.

4.Boredom and Lack of Purpose: Feeling unfulfilled or without direction can cause individuals to seek comfort in food.

5.Social and Cultural Pressures: Societal beauty standards, media influences, and cultural expectations can contribute to emotional eating.

Signs of Emotional Eating

1.Eating in Secret: Hiding food or eating alone to avoid judgment or shame.

2.Using Food as a Reward or Punishment: Treating yourself with food for accomplishments or using food to cope with guilt or shame.

3.Eating When Not Hungry: Consuming food in response to emotional cues, rather than physical hunger.

4.Feeling Guilty or Ashamed After Eating: Experiencing negative emotions after consuming food, leading to a cycle of self-criticism.

5.Using Food to Cope with Emotions: Turning to food to manage stress, anxiety, or other emotions.

Consequences of Emotional Eating

1.Weight Gain and Obesity: Consuming excess calories and unhealthy foods can lead to weight gain and obesity.

2.Nutrient Imbalance: Regularly eating processed and high-calorie foods can result in nutrient deficiencies and poor overall health.

3.Mental Health Issues: Emotional eating can exacerbate existing mental health conditions, such as depression and anxiety.

4.Social Isolation: Shame and guilt associated with emotional eating can lead to social withdrawal and isolation.

5.Lack of Self-Care: Neglecting self-care and prioritizing food over well-being can result in burnout and decreased self-esteem.

Breaking the Cycle of Emotional Eating

1.Recognize Your Emotional Triggers: Identify the emotions that drive your eating.

2.Pause and Reflect: Before eating, take a moment to assess your emotional state.

3.Find Healthy Coping Mechanisms: Replace food with alternative coping strategies, such as:

- Deep breathing   - Exercise
- Journaling
- Creative activities
- Social support

4.Develop a Self-Care Plan: Prioritize self-care activities to manage stress and emotions.

5.Practice Mindful Eating: Savor your food, pay attention to hunger and fullness cues, and eat slowly.

6.Seek Support: Share your struggles with a trusted friend, family member, or mental health professional.

Strategies for Overcoming Emotional Eating

1.Keep a Food and Mood Journal: Record your eating habits and emotional state to identify patterns.

2.Develop a Healthy Relationship with Food: Focus on nourishment, rather than comfort.

3.Find Healthy Ways to Celebrate:
Replace food with alternative celebration
methods, such as:
   - Activities (e.g., hiking, painting)
    - Social connections (e.g., phone calls,
outings)
    - Personal growth (e.g., learning a new
skill)

4.Practice Self-Compassion: Treat yourself
with kindness and understanding, rather than
judgment.

**5.Gradually Exposure Yourself to
Emotional Situations:** Build resilience by
gradually facing situations that trigger
emotional eating.

Here's a sample plan to help you overcome emotional eating:

Monday

- Identify emotional triggers (journaling)
- Practise deep breathing exercises (5
minutes)

Tuesday

- Engage in a creative activity (30 minutes)
- Reflect on emotional state before eating (pause and reflect)

Wednesday

- Exercise (30 minutes)
- Connect with a friend or family member (social support)

Thursday

- Practise mindful eating (slow, savoring)
- Develop a self-care plan (schedule self-care activities)

Friday

- Keep a food and mood journal (record eating habits and emotional state)
- Find healthy ways to celebrate (alternative celebration methods)

Saturday

- Engage in a relaxing activity (e.g., yoga, reading)
- Practise self-compassion (treat yourself with kindness)

Sunday

- Gradually expose yourself to emotional situations (build resilience)
- Reflect on progress and challenges (journaling)

Remember, overcoming emotional eating takes time, patience, and self-awareness. Be gentle with yourself, and don't hesitate to seek support when needed. By breaking the cycle of emotional eating, you'll develop a healthier relationship with food and your emotions.

Chapter 7:

Building a Supportive Community

Having a supportive community is crucial for achieving success and maintaining motivation on your weight loss journey. Surrounding yourself with like-minded individuals who understand your struggles and goals can provide encouragement, accountability, and a sense of belonging. In this chapter, we'll explore ways to build a supportive community that will help you stay on track and reach your goals.

Why a Supportive Community

1.Accountability: A supportive community provides a sense of responsibility, helping you stay committed to your goals.

2.Encouragement: Surrounding yourself with positive and supportive individuals boosts motivation and confidence.

3.Shared Experiences: Connecting with others who face similar challenges creates a sense of camaraderie and understanding.

4.Diverse Perspectives:A supportive community offers varying viewpoints and advice, helping you find solutions to obstacles.

5.Celebrating Successes: Sharing achievements with a supportive community amplifies joy and reinforces progress.

Ways to Build a Supportive Community

1.Join Online Forums or Social Media Groups: Connect with others through online platforms focused on weight loss and wellness.

2.Attend Local Support Groups or Meetups: Participate in in-person gatherings, such as weight loss support groups or fitness classes.

3.Find a Workout Buddy or Accountability Partner: Share your goals and progress with a friend or family member and ask them to hold you accountable.

4.Participate in Online Challenges or Events: Engage in virtual events, such as fitness challenges or webinars, to connect with others and stay motivated.

5.Volunteer or Help Others: Assist others in their weight loss journeys, providing support and guidance while strengthening your own commitment.

Tips for Nurturing Your Supportive Community

1.Be Open and Honest: Share your struggles and successes with your community, fostering trust and empathy.

2.Listen and Offer Support: Provide encouragement and guidance to others, just as you would like to receive.

3.Respect and Celebrate Differences: Embrace diverse perspectives and goals within your community.

4.Stay Consistent and Patient: Understand that progress may vary, and be patient with yourself and others.

5.Lead by Example: Demonstrate positive habits and a growth mindset, inspiring others to do the same.

By building a supportive community, you'll create a network of individuals who understand your journey and can offer valuable guidance, encouragement, and motivation. Remember, having a supportive community is crucial for long-term success, so nurture and cherish these relationships.

Chapter 8:

Maintaining Progress and Celebrating Success

Congratulations on reaching this milestone! You've worked hard to achieve your weight loss goals, and now it's time to focus on maintaining progress and celebrating your success. In this chapter, we'll explore strategies for sustaining your weight loss journey and acknowledging your accomplishments.

Maintaining Progress

1.**Set New Goals:** Continue challenging yourself with new, achievable goals to maintain motivation.

2.**Monitor Progress:** Regularly track your weight, measurements, and progress photos to stay aware of your progress.

3.Stay Hydrated and Nutrient-Dense: Continue prioritizing healthy eating habits and adequate hydration.

4.Incorporate Variety in Your Routine: Mix up your workout routine and try new activities to avoid plateaus.

5.Get Enough Sleep and Manage Stress: Prioritize restful sleep and effective stress management techniques.

Celebrating Success

1.Acknowledge Your Achievements: Recognize and celebrate your hard work and dedication.

2.Treat Yourself: Indulge in non-food related rewards, like a relaxing bath or a fun activity.

3.Share Your Success: Inspire others by sharing your journey and progress on social media or with friends and family.

4.Reflect on Your Journey: Write down your experiences, lessons learned, and how far you've come.

5.Continue Learning and Growing: Stay informed about new health and wellness trends, and incorporate them into your lifestyle.

Tips for Long-Term Success

1.Be Patient and Persistent: Maintaining a healthy weight loss journey requires patience and persistence. It's necessary that you understand that progress may not always be linear, and setbacks are a natural part of the process. Here are some tips to help you cultivate patience and persistence:

Focus on Progress, Not Perfection: Recognize that small steps lead to significant changes over time.

Celebrate Small Victories: Acknowledge and celebrate your achievements, no matter how small they may seem.

Embrace the Journey: View your weight loss journey as a long-term investment in your health and well-being.

Don't Obsess Over Scales: Focus on how you feel, rather than just the number on the scale.

Practice Mindfulness: Stay present and focused on the current moment, rather than worrying about the future or past.

Persistence

Set Realistic Goals: Break your goals into smaller, achievable milestones to maintain motivation.

Create a Support System: Surround yourself with people who encourage and support your journey.

Find Healthy Coping Mechanisms: Develop strategies to manage stress and emotions, rather than turning to food.

Learn from Setbacks: Use setbacks as opportunities to learn and grow, rather than giving up.

Stay Consistent: Make healthy habits a part of your daily routine, even when it feels challenging.

2.Embrace Self-Care: Prioritise activities that nourish your mind, body, and spirit.
Self-care is an essential aspect of maintaining a healthy weight loss journey. It involves nurturing your overall well-being, including your physical, mental, and emotional health. By prioritising self-care, you'll become more resilient, confident, and better equipped to handle challenges. Here are some ways to embrace self-care:

Physical Self-Care

Get Enough Sleep: Aim for 7-9 hours of restful sleep per night to help regulate hunger hormones and support weight loss.

Stay Hydrated: Drink plenty of water throughout the day to help control hunger and boost energy.

Engage in Gentle Exercise: Incorporate low-impact activities like yoga, walking, or swimming to promote relaxation and flexibility.

Practice Good Hygiene: Take care of your physical appearance to boost confidence and self-esteem.

Mental and Emotional Self-Care

Meditate and Practice Mindfulness: Regularly take a few minutes to focus on your breath, calm your mind, and reduce stress.

Write in a Journal: Express your thoughts, feelings, and gratitudes to process emotions and gain insight.

Connect with Nature: Spend time outdoors, whether walking, gardening, or simply sitting in a park or backyard.

Engage in Creative Activities: Explore hobbies like painting, drawing, writing, or photography to tap into your creativity and relaxation.

Emotional Self-Care

Set Healthy Boundaries: Learn to say "no" and prioritize your needs without feeling guilty.

Practice Self-Compassion: Treat yourself with kindness, understanding, and patience, just as you would a close friend.

Seek Support: Surround yourself with positive, supportive people who encourage and uplift you.

Take Breaks and Prioritize Relaxation: Allow yourself time to rest and recharge, without feeling guilty or selfish.

3.Stay Positive and Focus on Progress:

Celebrate small victories and acknowledge your growth.
Maintaining a positive mindset and focusing on progress is crucial for a successful weight loss journey. It helps you stay motivated, encouraged, and committed to your goals.

Here are some tips to help you stay positive and focused on progress:

Reframe Negative Thoughts: Challenge negative self-talk by replacing critical inner voices with positive affirmations.

Celebrate Small Wins: Acknowledge and celebrate small victories along the way, like a healthy meal or a good workout.

Focus on Progress,Not Perfection: Embrace the journey and focus on progress, rather than expecting immediate perfection.

Practice Gratitude: Reflect on the things you're thankful for, like good health, supportive friends, or a comfortable home.

Surround Yourself with Positivity: Seek out encouraging people, inspiring stories, and uplifting environments.

Take Care of Your Mental Health_: Prioritize stress management, self-care, and emotional well-being.

Embrace the Process: View your weight loss journey as a transformative experience, rather than just a destination.

Stay Present: Focus on the present moment and what you can control, rather than worrying about the future or past.

Find the Lesson: When faced with setbacks, seek out the lesson or opportunity for growth.

Smile and Laugh Often: Cultivate joy and positivity by smiling and laughing regularly.

4.Seek Support When Needed:
Seeking support when needed is a crucial aspect of maintaining a healthy weight loss journey. It's essential to recognize that you don't have to do it alone and that asking for help is a sign of strength, not weakness. Here are some ways to seek support when needed:

Friends and Family: Share your goals and progress with trusted friends and family members and ask for their encouragement and support.

Support Groups: Join online or in-person support groups, like Weight Watchers or Overeaters Anonymous, to connect with others who share similar goals and challenges.

Mentor or Coach: Work with a health coach, nutritionist, or personal trainer who can provide guidance, accountability, and motivation.

Online Communities: Participate in online forums, social media groups, or blogs focused on weight loss and wellness to connect with others and find support.

Professional Help: If struggling with emotional eating, disordered eating, or other mental health concerns, consider seeking help from a mental health professional.

Accountability Partner: Find someone who shares similar goals and schedule regular check-ins to track progress and offer support.

Hotlines and Resources: Utilize resources like the National Eating Disorders Association (NEDA) hotline or the

Academy of Nutrition and Dietetics for guidance and support.

Self-Care Professionals: Work with professionals like therapists, counselors, or life coaches to address underlying issues and develop coping strategies.

Supportive Healthcare Providers: Find healthcare providers who support and encourage your weight loss journey.

Be Open and Honest: Don't be afraid to ask for help when needed and be open and honest about your struggles and progress.

Remember, seeking support when needed is a sign of strength and can make a significant difference in your weight loss journey. Don't be afraid to reach out and ask for help – you don't have to do it alone!

5.Keep a Growth Mindset: Embrace new experiences and view challenges as opportunities for growth.

By implementing these strategies, you'll maintain your progress and continue celebrating your success. Remember, your weight loss journey is a long-term commitment to your health and well-being. Stay dedicated, patient, and kind to yourself, and you'll achieve lasting success.

Conclusion

Congratulations on completing this comprehensive guide to achieving a healthy weight loss journey! You've learned the importance of:

1. Setting realistic goals: Break down your goals into smaller, achievable milestones to maintain motivation and track progress.

2. Creating a supportive environment: Surround yourself with positive influences, remove unhealthy temptations, and establish a routine that promotes healthy habits.

3. Developing a positive mindset: Focus on progress, not perfection, and cultivate self-awareness, self-compassion, and self-forgiveness.

4. Overcoming emotional eating: Identify triggers, practice mindful eating, and develop healthy coping mechanisms to manage emotions.

5. Building a supportive community: Join online forums, attend support groups, or find

an accountability partner to share experiences and receive encouragement.

6. Maintaining progress: Stay consistent, celebrate small victories, and be patient with setbacks to ensure long-term success.

Always keep in mind, weight loss is not just about physical transformation; it's also about mental and emotional growth. By focusing on progress, not perfection, and seeking support when needed, you'll cultivate a resilient mindset and achieve long-term success.

As you continue on your weight loss journey, keep in mind the following final tips:

- Be patient and kind to yourself: Treat yourself with the same kindness and compassion you offer to others.

- Focus on progress, not perfection: Celebrate small victories and acknowledge the journey, rather than fixating on the destination.

- Seek support when needed: Don't hesitate to ask for help when facing challenges or setbacks.

- Celebrate small victories: Acknowledge and celebrate milestones, no matter how small they may seem.

- Stay committed to your goals: Stay dedicated to your goals, even when faced with obstacles or temptations.

You are capable of achieving a healthy weight loss journey. Believe in yourself, stay committed, and celebrate your progress along the way!

www.ingramcontent.com/pod-product-compliance
Lightning Source LLC
Chambersburg PA
CBHW071045250726
48653CB00005B/2013